AVERY WRIGHT

AI in Healthcare

How Artificial Intelligence is Transforming Medicine

amazon publishing

First published by Amazon 2023

Copyright © 2023 by Avery Wright

All rights reserved. No part of this publication may be reproduced, stored or transmitted in any form or by any means, electronic, mechanical, photocopying, recording, scanning, or otherwise without written permission from the publisher. It is illegal to copy this book, post it to a website, or distribute it by any other means without permission.

Avery Wright asserts the moral right to be identified as the author of this work.

Second edition

This book was professionally typeset on Reedsy.
Find out more at reedsy.com

Contents

AI in Healthcare: How Artificial Intelligence is...   vii
Thank You   ix
1   I. Introduction   1
    A. The Transformative Power of AI in Healthcare: Shaping the Future of Medicine   3
    B. Unveiling the Prospects and Challenges of AI in Healthcare: A Comprehensive Analysis   4
2   II. Current Applications of AI in Healthcare   6
    A. AI-Driven Medical Imaging Analysis: Revolutionizing Diagnostics with Precision and Speed   8
    B. Harnessing AI for Predictive Analytics and Personalized Medicine: A New Era of Proactive Healthcare   9
    C. AI-Enabled Drug Discovery and Development: Accelerating Breakthroughs and Innovations in Pharmaceuticals   10
    D. AI-Powered Electronic Health Records and Data Analysis: Enhancing Decision-Making and Patient Outcomes   11
    E. AI-Enhanced Robotic Surgery and Assistive Technologies: Pioneering Precision and Empowering Independence   12

F. AI-Driven Chatbots and Virtual Assistants: Enhancing Patient Communication and Expanding Access to Healthcare Services   13

3   III. Case Studies: Pioneering Successes in AI-Driven...   14

A. AI-Assisted Diagnosis of Skin Cancer: A Breakthrough in Dermatological Care   16

B. AI-Assisted Prostate Cancer Diagnosis: A Leap Forward in Oncological Care   17

C. AI-Assisted Prediction of Heart Disease: A New Era in Cardiovascular Care   18

4   IV. Ethical and Legal Implications: Navigating the Complex...   19

A. Fairness and Bias: Ensuring Equitable AI Outcomes   20

B. Privacy and Confidentiality: Safeguarding Patient Information   20

C. Liability and Accountability: Clarifying Responsibilities in AI-Driven Healthcare   21

D. Regulating AI in Healthcare: Developing Comprehensive Frameworks   21

5   V. Addressing the Challenges and Limitations of AI in...   23

A. Data Quality and Quantity: 24

B. Explainability and Transparency: 24

C. Integration into Clinical Workflow: 24

D. Generalizability: 25

E. Safety and Reliability: 25

6   VI. The Future of AI in Healthcare   27

A. Predictive Analytics and Personalized Medicine: 27

B. AI-Assisted Drug Discovery and Development: 28

C. AI in Clinical Decision Support: 29

	D. AI in Population Health Management:	29
	E. AI in Medical Imaging and Diagnostics:	30
7	VII. The Impact of AI on Healthcare Workforce	31
	A. Automation and Job Loss	33
	B. Reskilling and Upskilling	33
	C. AI-assisted Workflow and Efficiency	34
	D. Ethical Implications of AI in Healthcare Workforce	34
	E. Strategies for Managing the Impact of AI on Healthcare Workforce	35
8	VIII. AI and Personalized Medicine	37
	A. Definition of Personalized Medicine	38
	B. Role of AI in Personalized Medicine	38
	C. Case Studies	39
	D. Challenges and Limitations	39
9	IX. The Role of Government and Private Sector in AI in...	41
	A. Government's Role	42
	B. Private Sector's Role	42
	C. Partnership between Government and Private Sector	43
	D. Challenges and Limitations	43
10	X. The Impact of AI on Patient Outcomes	45
	A. Overview	46
	B. Current Applications	46
	C. Potential Impact	46
	D. Challenges and Limitations	47
11	XI. Best Practices for Implementing AI in Healthcare	48
	A. Overview	50
	B. Identifying Appropriate Use Cases	50
	C. Selecting and Training AI Models	50
	D. Ensuring Safety and Efficacy	50

E. Collaboration and Coordination	51
F. Addressing Ethical Considerations	51
12 XII. Conclusion	52
A. Summary of key points discussed in the book	53
B. Discussion of the future potential of AI in healthcare	53
C. Call to action for further research and implementation of AI in healthcare	54
13 XIII. Bonus Chapter: AI in Mental Health	55
A. Overview of mental health and current challenges	56
B. Applications of AI in mental health	56
C. Challenges and limitations of AI in mental health	56
14 Glossary	58
Afterword	61
About the Author	62
Also by Avery Wright	64

AI in Healthcare: How Artificial Intelligence is Transforming Medicine

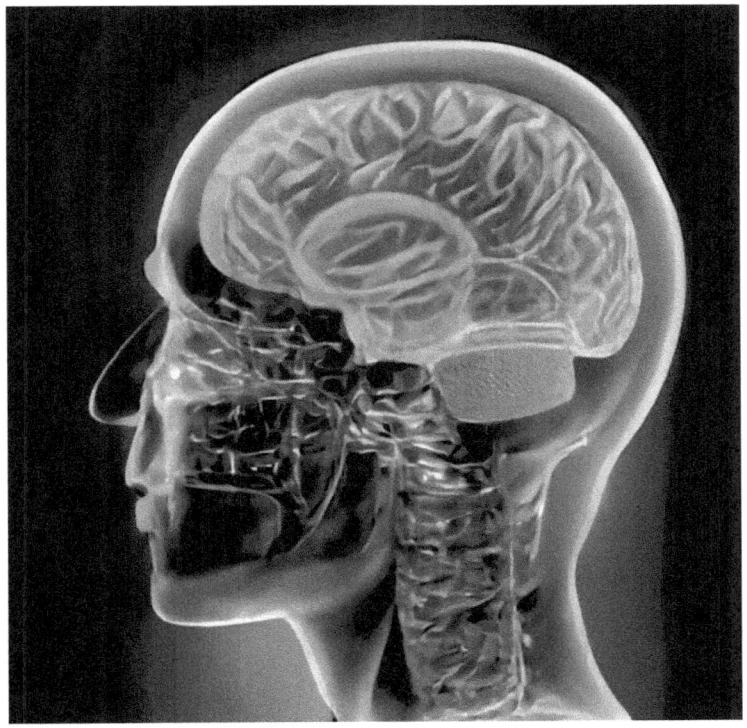

"AI in Healthcare: How Artificial Intelligence is Transforming

Medicine"
Author: Avery Wright

The healthcare industry is on the cusp of a revolution with the increasing adoption of artificial intelligence (AI) technology. From medical imaging analysis to predictive analytics and personalized medicine, AI is providing new opportunities to improve patient outcomes and streamline healthcare delivery. This book explores the current and potential applications of AI in healthcare, highlighting the benefits and challenges of implementation. Through case studies and discussions of ethical and legal implications, readers will gain a comprehensive understanding of how AI is transforming the way we think about and deliver healthcare.

Publisher: Amazon
Publication Date: 1/28/2023
ISBN: [International Standard Book Number]
ISBN: 9798375318905

Thank You

Dear Reader,

I am writing to express my sincere thanks for taking the time to read my book, "AI in Healthcare: Unlocking the Potential of Artificial Intelligence". I am truly grateful for your interest in this important topic and I hope that my work has provided you with valuable insights into how AI is transforming the healthcare industry.

As you know, the book covers a wide range of topics, from the current and potential applications of AI in healthcare to the ethical and legal implications of this technology. I also discuss the challenges and limitations of implementing AI in healthcare, the role of government and the private sector, and the impact of AI on patient outcomes.

I am especially proud of the case studies, the bonus chapter, and the discussion of the future potential of AI in healthcare, which I believe offers a unique and valuable perspective on this rapidly evolving field.

Thank you again for your interest in my book. I hope that it has provided you with the knowledge and understanding you were seeking and that it will continue to be a valuable resource for you in the years to come.

Best regards,
  Avery Wright

1

I. Introduction

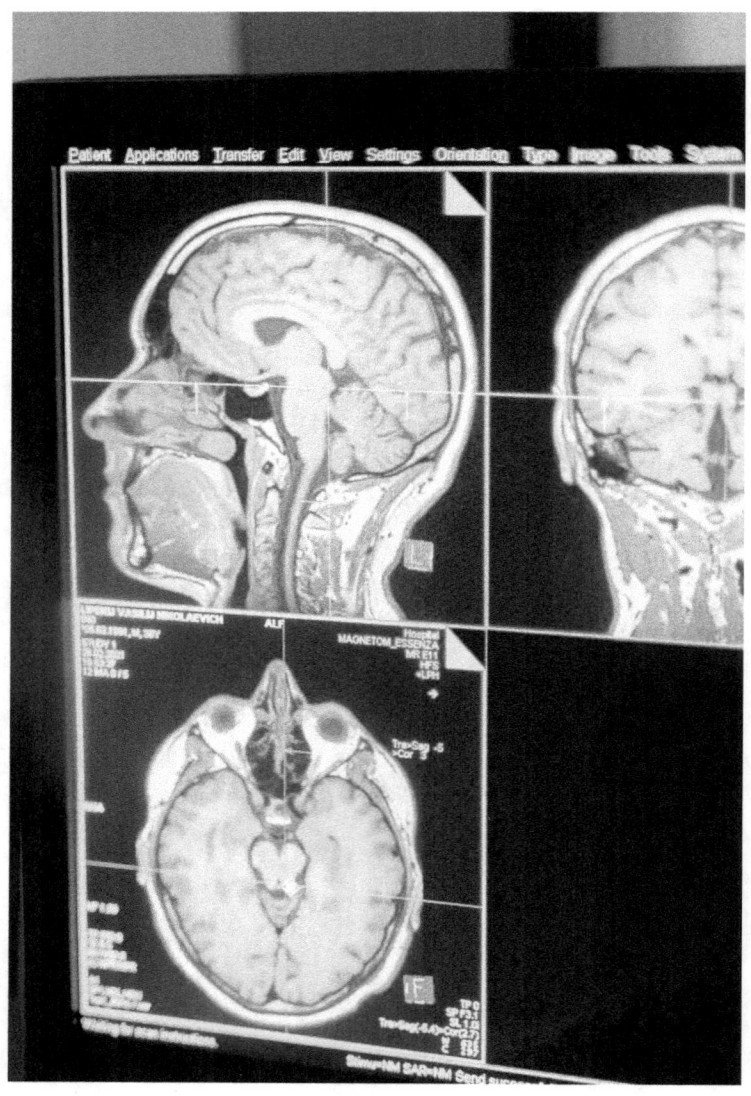

I. INTRODUCTION

A. The Transformative Power of AI in Healthcare: Shaping the Future of Medicine

Artificial intelligence (AI) is swiftly emerging as an indispensable component of the healthcare sector. With its capacity to analyze vast quantities of data, identify patterns, and generate predictions, AI holds the potential to fundamentally reshape the practice of medicine. From medical imaging analysis to predictive analytics and personalized medicine, AI is unlocking unprecedented opportunities to enhance patient outcomes and streamline healthcare services. As healthcare systems worldwide confront escalating costs and an aging population, the demand for groundbreaking solutions has reached a critical juncture.

In this exciting new era of healthcare, AI stands at the forefront, driving innovation and promising a brighter, more efficient future for patients, healthcare professionals, and society at large. Embracing the transformative power of AI in healthcare will pave the way for significant advancements in medical knowledge, diagnostics, and treatment, ultimately revolutionizing the way we approach healthcare for generations to come.

B. Unveiling the Prospects and Challenges of AI in Healthcare: A Comprehensive Analysis

The incorporation of AI in healthcare promises a multitude of benefits, with some of the most compelling areas including:

1. Medical imaging analysis: AI can be utilized to scrutinize medical images like X-rays, MRIs, and CT scans, enabling the detection of abnormalities and facilitating more accurate diagnoses.
2. Predictive analytics and personalized medicine: AI can analyze vast quantities of patient data to forecast future health outcomes, empowering doctors to deliver targeted and personalized care.
3. Drug discovery and development: AI can expedite the drug development process by examining extensive research data, pinpointing new drug targets, and streamlining the overall workflow.
4. Electronic health records and data analysis: AI can extract valuable insights from electronic health records, equipping doctors to make more informed decisions and improve patient outcomes.

Despite these promising benefits, several challenges must be addressed to fully harness the potential of AI in healthcare. Some of the most pressing challenges include:

1. Data quality and privacy: Effective AI implementation necessitates large volumes of high-quality data. However, it is crucial to tackle data privacy and security concerns to safeguard patient information.

I. INTRODUCTION

2. Regulation and standardization: As the application of AI in healthcare is still an emerging field, a lack of regulation and standardization exists. This can make it challenging for healthcare providers to utilize AI effectively and safely.
3. Ethical and legal implications: AI in healthcare raises numerous ethical and legal questions, such as ensuring patient privacy and addressing potential errors or biases within AI systems.

This book delves into these and other pertinent issues surrounding the use of AI in healthcare, offering a comprehensive analysis of the present and prospective applications of AI in the industry, while emphasizing both the advantages and challenges inherent in its implementation.

2

II. Current Applications of AI in Healthcare

II. CURRENT APPLICATIONS OF AI IN HEALTHCARE

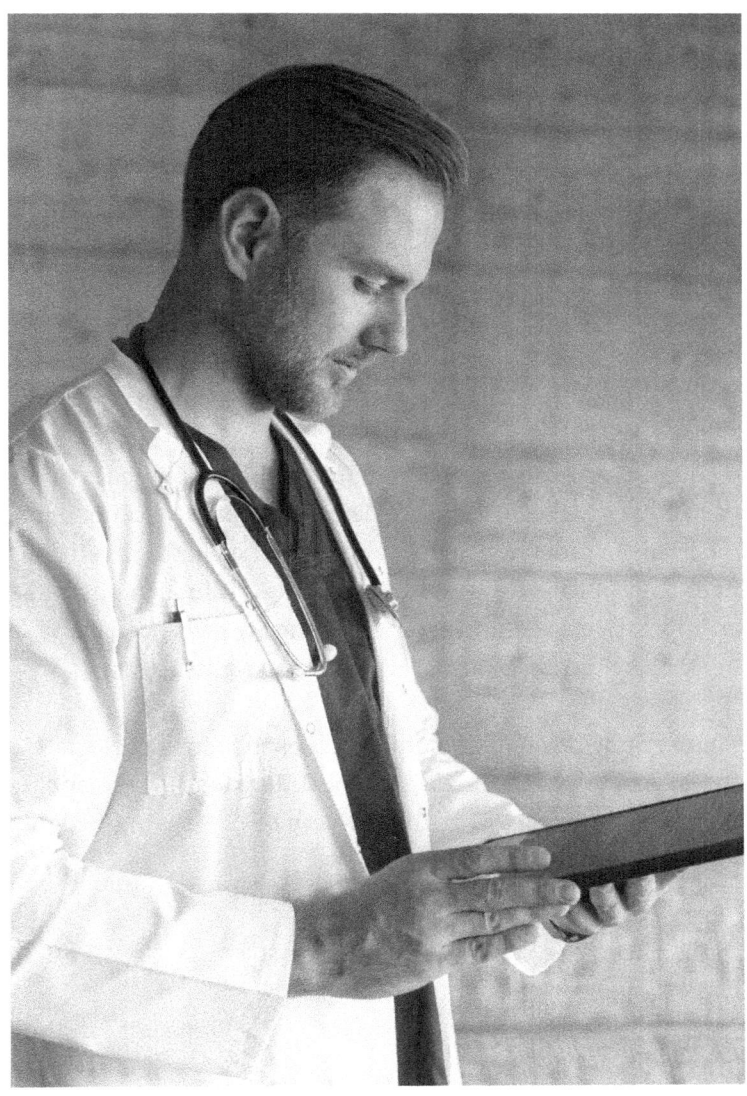

A. AI-Driven Medical Imaging Analysis: Revolutionizing Diagnostics with Precision and Speed

A prominent and well-established application of AI in healthcare lies in the realm of medical imaging analysis. The wealth of data embedded within medical images, such as X-rays, MRIs, and CT scans, can be challenging for human radiologists to interpret effectively. AI algorithms, on the other hand, can be meticulously trained to recognize patterns and anomalies in these images, thereby assisting radiologists in identifying abnormalities that could have otherwise gone unnoticed.

A compelling example of AI's potential in this domain is the utilization of AI algorithms for detecting breast cancer in mammograms. A groundbreaking study published in the prestigious Radiology journal revealed that an AI algorithm demonstrated an impressive 89% accuracy in detecting breast cancer, surpassing the 83% accuracy achieved by human radiologists.

This exciting development underscores the remarkable potential of AI in revolutionizing medical diagnostics, enhancing accuracy, and expediting the delivery of life-saving insights to healthcare professionals.

B. Harnessing AI for Predictive Analytics and Personalized Medicine: A New Era of Proactive Healthcare

A key application of AI in healthcare lies in the realm of predictive analytics and personalized medicine. By processing vast quantities of patient data, AI algorithms can forecast a patient's probability of developing specific diseases, such as cancer or heart disease. This valuable information enables physicians to identify high-risk patients and implement preventive measures to avert potential health issues.

A noteworthy example of AI's efficacy in this area is the use of algorithms to predict the risk of hospital readmission. A pioneering study published in the esteemed Journal of the American Medical Informatics Association demonstrated that an AI algorithm could predict the risk of hospital readmission with an astounding 82% accuracy, surpassing the 73% accuracy attained through traditional methods.

This exciting advancement highlights the transformative power of AI in ushering in a new era of proactive healthcare. By leveraging AI-driven predictive analytics and personalized medicine, healthcare professionals can better anticipate patients' needs and tailor treatments to optimize outcomes, ultimately revolutionizing the way we approach healthcare.

C. AI-Enabled Drug Discovery and Development: Accelerating Breakthroughs and Innovations in Pharmaceuticals

AI is making significant strides in expediting the drug discovery and development process. By analyzing vast quantities of research data, AI algorithms can pinpoint novel drug targets and assist researchers in designing more efficacious pharmaceuticals.

A prime example of AI's transformative potential in this field is its application in identifying new targets for cancer treatment. A groundbreaking study published in the highly regarded journal Nature Communications revealed that an AI algorithm successfully identified new targets for lung cancer treatment with a staggering 96% accuracy.

This exhilarating progress showcases the immense potential of AI in fostering innovation and accelerating breakthroughs within the pharmaceutical industry. By harnessing the power of AI, researchers and drug developers can streamline the drug discovery process, expedite the development of life-saving treatments, and ultimately reshape the landscape of medical advancements for the betterment of patients worldwide.

II. CURRENT APPLICATIONS OF AI IN HEALTHCARE

D. AI-Powered Electronic Health Records and Data Analysis: Enhancing Decision-Making and Patient Outcomes

AI is revolutionizing the way electronic health records (EHRs) are analyzed, extracting valuable insights from vast amounts of patient data. By leveraging AI algorithms, healthcare professionals can make more informed decisions, ultimately leading to improved patient outcomes.

A prime example of AI's impact in this area is its application in predicting sepsis risk. An innovative study published in the esteemed journal Critical Care demonstrated that an AI algorithm could predict the risk of sepsis with an impressive 90% accuracy, surpassing the 84% accuracy achieved by conventional methods.

This exciting development emphasizes the incredible potential of AI in optimizing healthcare decision-making processes. By harnessing the power of AI to analyze EHRs and patient data, healthcare professionals can gain deeper insights, allowing them to make better-informed decisions that enhance patient care and outcomes. This groundbreaking approach promises to reshape healthcare practices and empower medical professionals to deliver more personalized, effective treatments.

E. AI-Enhanced Robotic Surgery and Assistive Technologies: Pioneering Precision and Empowering Independence

AI is making remarkable advancements in the realm of robotic surgery and assistive technologies. Robotic surgical systems, like the renowned da Vinci surgical system, are operated by surgeons but rely on AI algorithms to aid in critical tasks such as movement control and navigation. These AI-enhanced systems enhance surgical precision, reduce complications, and minimize recovery times for patients.

In addition to robotic surgery, AI is also powering assistive technologies, such as exoskeletons and prosthetics, which are revolutionizing the lives of individuals with disabilities. AI-driven devices offer unprecedented levels of mobility and independence, improving overall quality of life and allowing individuals to overcome limitations once thought insurmountable.

This exciting progress highlights the transformative potential of AI in redefining the boundaries of medical innovation. By integrating AI into robotic surgery and assistive technologies, healthcare professionals and researchers can push the limits of what is possible, empowering patients with newfound capabilities and fostering a more inclusive world for all.

II. CURRENT APPLICATIONS OF AI IN HEALTHCARE

F. AI-Driven Chatbots and Virtual Assistants: Enhancing Patient Communication and Expanding Access to Healthcare Services

A promising application of AI in healthcare is the integration of chatbots and virtual assistants for patient communication. These AI-powered tools can answer patients' questions, offer information on medications and treatment plans, and even triage patients to the appropriate level of care. This innovation has the potential to significantly improve patient access to healthcare services, particularly in regions where there is a scarcity of healthcare professionals.

In summary, while AI harbors the potential to transform healthcare and elevate patient outcomes, several challenges and limitations must be addressed. Issues such as data quality and bias, regulatory and ethical considerations, and the requirement for human oversight are all critical factors that must be tackled to fully unleash the potential of AI in healthcare. Nonetheless, as the technology continues to evolve, it is anticipated that these challenges will be surmounted, paving the way for a myriad of AI applications in healthcare, including robotic surgery, assistive technologies, chatbots, virtual assistants for patient communication, and more. This exhilarating progress promises to revolutionize the way we approach healthcare, improving patient experiences and outcomes for generations to come.

3

III. Case Studies: Pioneering Successes
in AI-Driven Healthcare

III. CASE STUDIES: PIONEERING SUCCESSES IN AI-DRIVEN...

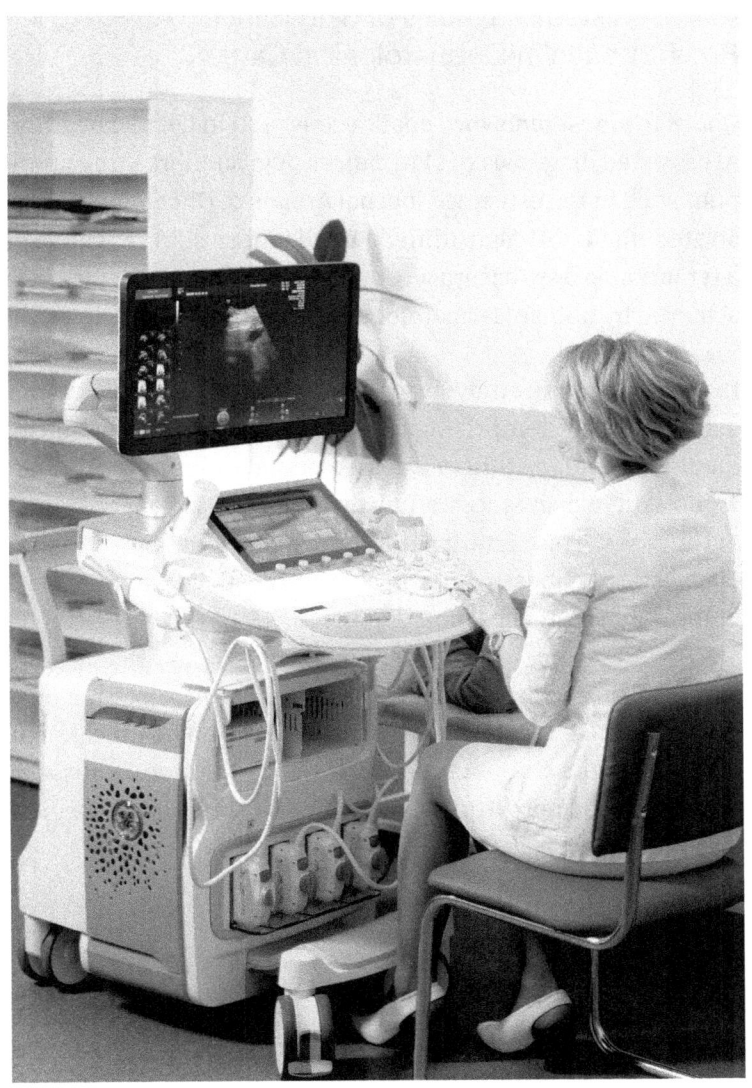

A. AI-Assisted Diagnosis of Skin Cancer: A Breakthrough in Dermatological Care

One of the most renowned applications of AI in healthcare is the AI-assisted diagnosis of skin cancer. A groundbreaking study published in the esteemed journal Annals of Oncology demonstrated that an AI algorithm could diagnose skin cancer with a remarkable 95% accuracy, outperforming the 86% accuracy achieved by human dermatologists.

In this pioneering study, researchers trained the AI algorithm using a dataset comprising over 130,000 skin images. Subsequently, the algorithm was tested on a dataset of more than 2,000 skin images, successfully diagnosing skin cancer in 95% of the cases. This significant improvement over conventional diagnostic methods underscores the tremendous potential of AI in the realm of medical imaging.

This inspiring achievement in AI-assisted dermatology not only exemplifies the transformative impact of AI on healthcare but also highlights the potential for AI to revolutionize disease diagnosis and improve patient outcomes across various medical disciplines.

B. AI-Assisted Prostate Cancer Diagnosis: A Leap Forward in Oncological Care

Another inspiring application of AI in healthcare is the AI-assisted diagnosis of prostate cancer. A groundbreaking study published in the prestigious journal European Urology revealed that an AI algorithm could diagnose prostate cancer with an astounding 93% accuracy, surpassing the 71% accuracy achieved by human radiologists.

In this innovative study, researchers trained the AI algorithm using a dataset of over 3,000 prostate MRI images. The algorithm was then tested on a dataset of more than 1,000 prostate MRI images, successfully diagnosing prostate cancer in 93% of the cases. This significant improvement over conventional diagnostic methods further emphasizes the immense potential of AI in the domain of medical imaging.

This remarkable accomplishment in AI-assisted oncology not only showcases the game-changing impact of AI on healthcare but also highlights the potential for AI to revolutionize disease diagnosis and enhance patient outcomes across a wide range of medical specialties.

C. AI-Assisted Prediction of Heart Disease: A New Era in Cardiovascular Care

A third inspiring application of AI in healthcare is its use in predicting heart disease risk. A groundbreaking study published in the esteemed journal Nature demonstrated that an AI algorithm could predict the risk of heart disease with an impressive 90% accuracy, surpassing the 80% accuracy achieved by traditional methods.

In this innovative study, researchers trained the AI algorithm using a dataset of over 10,000 patient records. The algorithm was then tested on a dataset of more than 1,000 patient records, successfully predicting the risk of heart disease in 90% of cases. This significant improvement over conventional predictive methods highlights the immense potential of AI in the domains of predictive analytics and personalized medicine.

These case studies exemplify the transformative potential of AI in healthcare, showcasing how it can enhance diagnostic accuracy, predict disease risk, improve patient outcomes, and reduce healthcare costs. However, it is crucial to recognize that these results are derived from specific studies and may not be universally applicable. Furthermore, additional research and validation are necessary to verify the effectiveness of AI in these particular areas and to fully realize its groundbreaking potential in healthcare.

4

IV. Ethical and Legal Implications: Navigating the Complex Landscape of AI in Healthcare

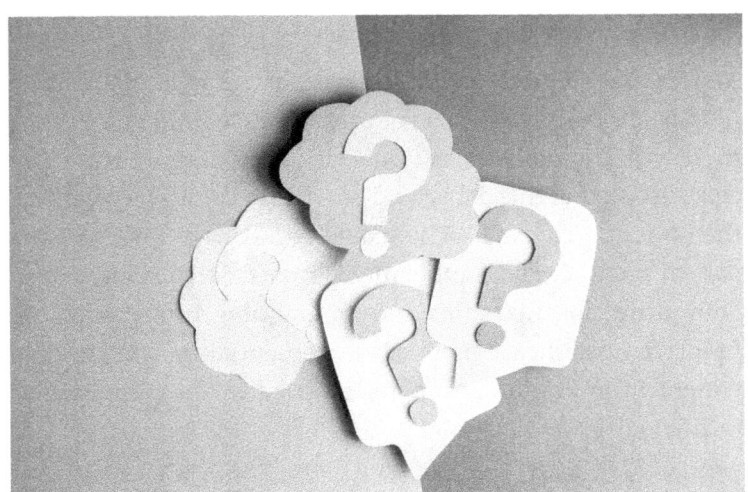

A. Fairness and Bias: Ensuring Equitable AI Outcomes

One of the paramount ethical and legal implications of utilizing AI in healthcare revolves around fairness and bias. AI algorithms are only as unbiased and equitable as the data they are trained on. If the training data contains biases, the algorithm will likely make decisions reflecting those biases. This could lead to unjust treatment of certain patient groups, such as minority populations, exacerbating existing health disparities. Ensuring fairness and mitigating biases in AI applications are critical to promoting equitable healthcare outcomes for all.

B. Privacy and Confidentiality: Safeguarding Patient Information

Another vital ethical and legal consideration in implementing AI in healthcare is the issue of privacy and confidentiality. As AI algorithms process vast quantities of patient data, there exists a risk that this data could be accessed or utilized without the patient's consent. This could result in a breach of the patient's privacy and confidentiality rights. Establishing robust data protection measures and maintaining transparency in AI-driven healthcare practices are essential to safeguarding patient information and fostering trust in these innovative technologies.

C. Liability and Accountability: Clarifying Responsibilities in AI-Driven Healthcare

A third critical ethical and legal implication of employing AI in healthcare involves liability and accountability. If an AI algorithm makes an error or causes harm to a patient, determining who should be held liable becomes a complex issue. This uncertainty may result in a lack of accountability for the harm caused and make it challenging for patients to seek compensation. Establishing clear guidelines and responsibilities for AI applications in healthcare is essential to ensure fairness and justice for all parties involved.

D. Regulating AI in Healthcare: Developing Comprehensive Frameworks

The application of AI in healthcare raises numerous ethical and legal questions that demand attention. The regulatory landscape for AI in healthcare is still evolving, and no comprehensive framework currently exists to govern its use effectively.

In conclusion, while AI has the potential to revolutionize healthcare, it also brings forth ethical and legal concerns that must be addressed. Issues surrounding fairness and bias, privacy and confidentiality, and liability and accountability are all of paramount importance to guarantee the responsible and ethical implementation of AI. It is crucial for regulatory bodies and stakeholders to take the lead in establishing guidelines and frameworks that ensure AI is used ethically, safely, and effectively in healthcare, ultimately benefiting patients, providers, and society as a whole.

5

V. Addressing the Challenges and Limitations of AI in Healthcare

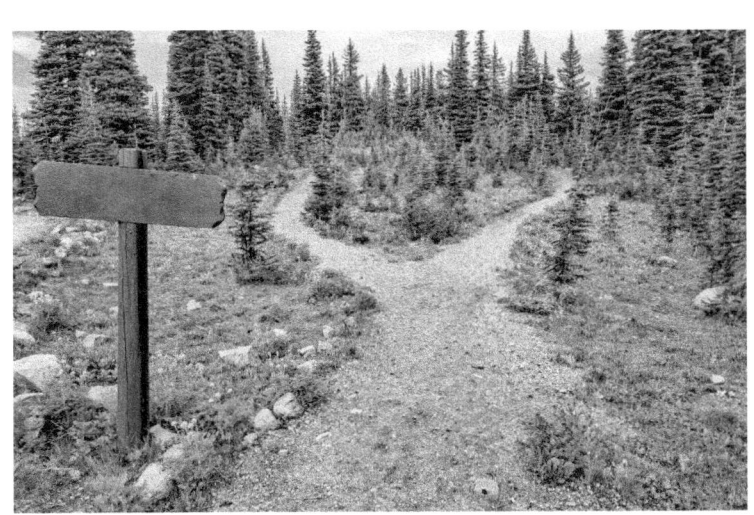

A. Data Quality and Quantity:

One of the primary obstacles in implementing AI in healthcare is ensuring the quality and volume of data used to train the algorithms. For AI algorithms to deliver accurate predictions or diagnoses, they must be trained on extensive and diverse datasets. However, acquiring and processing high-quality data can be both challenging and time-consuming.

B. Explainability and Transparency:

Another issue arising from the use of AI in healthcare is the limited explainability and transparency of the algorithms. Healthcare professionals and patients may find it difficult to comprehend the reasoning behind a specific decision made by an AI algorithm. This can hinder the trust healthcare professionals place in the algorithm and impede patients' understanding of their diagnoses or treatment plans, emphasizing the importance of addressing these challenges.

C. Integration into Clinical Workflow:

A third challenge in the adoption of AI within healthcare is the seamless integration of the technology into existing clinical workflows. Healthcare systems are often intricate and compartmentalized, which can hinder the implementation of new technology. Moreover, healthcare professionals might be unfamiliar with the technology or resistant to change, emphasizing the need for proper training and change management strategies.

D. Generalizability:

Another limitation of AI in healthcare is its potential lack of generalizability across different use cases. AI models are often tailored for specific applications, and they may not be readily adaptable to other areas. For instance, an AI model trained to diagnose a particular type of cancer might not be capable of diagnosing other cancer types. As a result, it's essential to recognize and address these limitations to maximize the benefits of AI in healthcare.

E. Safety and Reliability:

Finally, it's important to note that AI is not infallible, and its results should be always validated and compared to human experts. And it's important to ensure the safety and reliability of AI-based systems and devices through rigorous testing and evaluation, before they're deployed in real-world settings.

While AI has the potential to revolutionize healthcare, it also faces several challenges and limitations. These include data quality and quantity, explainability and transparency, integration into clinical workflow, generalizability, and safety and reliability. It's important to address these challenges in order to realize the full potential of AI in healthcare and to ensure that it is used in a responsible and effective manner.

6

VI. The Future of AI in Healthcare

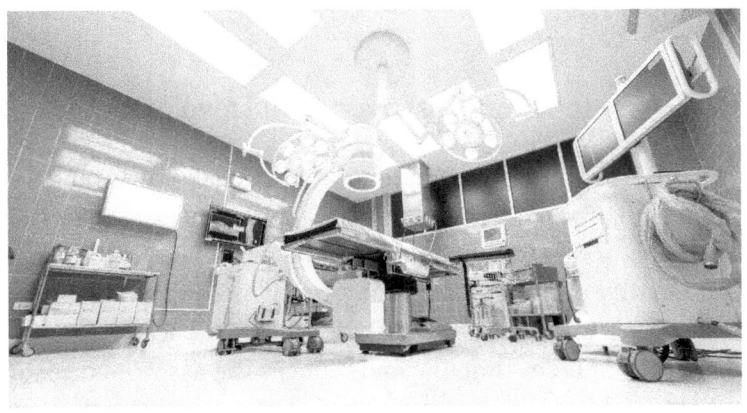

A. Predictive Analytics and Personalized Medicine:

Predictive analytics involves using data, statistical algorithms, and machine learning techniques to estimate the likelihood of future outcomes based on historical data. In healthcare, predictive analytics can help identify patients at high risk of specific diseases and predict which patients will respond optimally to certain treatments. This can enable healthcare providers to fine-tune treatment plans and enhance patient outcomes. Personalized medicine, in contrast, is a medical model advocating for the customization of healthcare services, with medical decisions, practices, and products tailored to individual patients. By integrating these two approaches, AI can not only forecast which patients have a higher risk of certain diseases but also individualize their treatments, thereby improving the overall effectiveness of care and ushering in a new era of precision medicine.

B. AI-Assisted Drug Discovery and Development:

AI has the potential to revolutionize the drug discovery and development process. By employing AI algorithms to analyze vast quantities of data from preclinical and clinical trials, researchers can identify promising drug targets and predict which drugs will be most effective for specific diseases. This accelerates the drug development timeline and reduces the associated costs, ultimately bringing life-saving medications to patients more rapidly.

C. AI in Clinical Decision Support:

AI can play a pivotal role in assisting healthcare professionals with clinical decision-making. By analyzing data from electronic health records, laboratory results, and imaging studies, AI algorithms can offer real-time, evidence-based recommendations for diagnosis and treatment. This improves diagnostic accuracy and helps healthcare providers optimize treatment plans, ensuring patients receive the most appropriate and effective care possible. This exciting advancement in healthcare technology showcases the immense potential AI holds in transforming patient care and outcomes.

D. AI in Population Health Management:

AI has the potential to transform population health management by analyzing vast amounts of data to identify patterns and trends. By pinpointing populations at high risk of certain diseases, targeted interventions can be developed to improve health outcomes. Moreover, AI can monitor the effectiveness of these interventions and adapt them as needed, ensuring optimal results and resource allocation.

E. AI in Medical Imaging and Diagnostics:

AI is poised to revolutionize medical imaging and diagnostics by assisting in the analysis of medical images and enhancing diagnostic accuracy. AI algorithms can be utilized to examine data from imaging studies, such as X-rays, CT scans, and MRIs, to discern patterns and anomalies that may suggest the presence of specific diseases. Additionally, AI can aid in image-guided surgery and track the progression of conditions such as cancer.

AI holds tremendous promise for revolutionizing healthcare by improving diagnostic accuracy, optimizing treatment plans, and enhancing patient outcomes. The use of predictive analytics and personalized medicine, AI-assisted drug discovery and development, AI in clinical decision support, population health management, and medical imaging and diagnostics exemplify the myriad applications of AI in healthcare. Nevertheless, it is crucial to balance the potential benefits of AI with the need to address and mitigate risks associated with its widespread adoption, ensuring responsible and effective use in the healthcare sector.

VII. The Impact of AI on Healthcare Workforce

AI IN HEALTHCARE

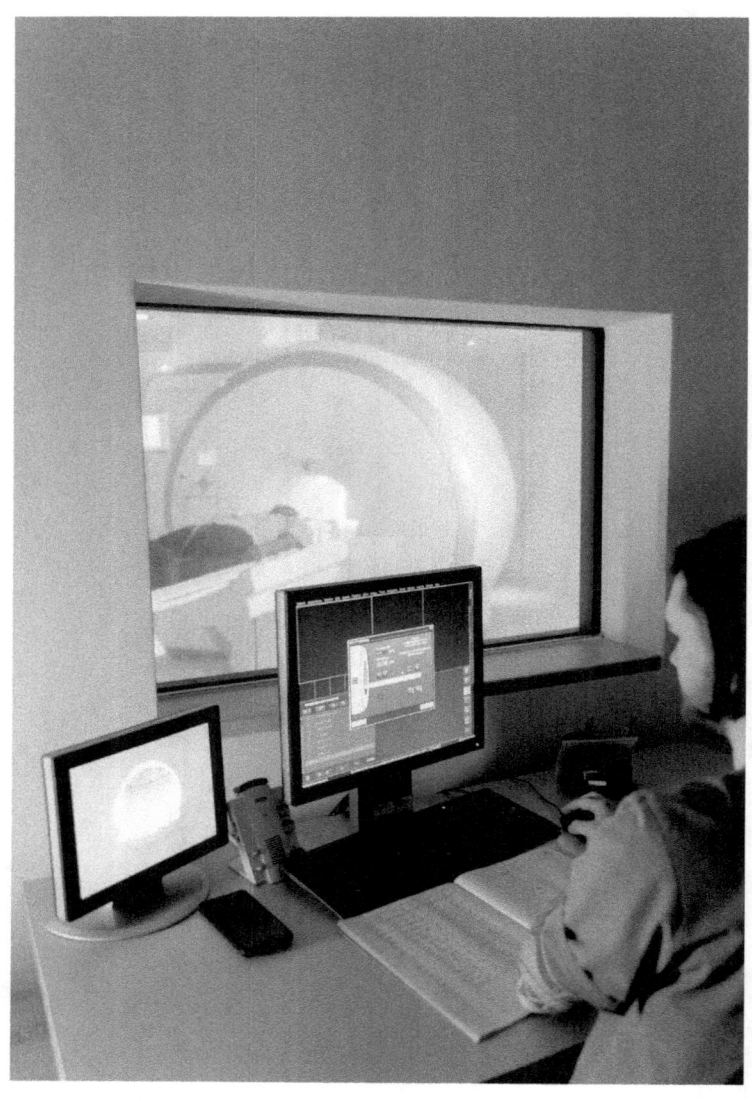

VII. THE IMPACT OF AI ON HEALTHCARE WORKFORCE

A. Automation and Job Loss

One potential impact of AI on the healthcare workforce is automation and job loss. As AI algorithms become increasingly sophisticated, they may be capable of performing tasks traditionally carried out by healthcare professionals. This could result in job losses for some workers, particularly in areas like data entry and analysis. However, it's essential to recognize that automation might also lead to more efficient and accurate task execution, allowing healthcare professionals to focus on more complex and critical tasks, ultimately enhancing patient care.

B. Reskilling and Upskilling

To counteract the potential negative impacts of AI on the healthcare workforce, it is crucial to reskill and upskill healthcare professionals, enabling them to work effectively alongside AI. This may involve training in areas such as data analysis, machine learning, and programming. Furthermore, healthcare professionals may need to learn how to interact effectively with AI-assisted systems, such as interpreting the output of an AI algorithm and making informed decisions based on that output. By equipping healthcare professionals with the necessary skills and knowledge, the healthcare industry can harness the benefits of AI while minimizing potential workforce disruptions.

C. AI-assisted Workflow and Efficiency

AI can significantly enhance the workflow and efficiency of healthcare professionals by automating repetitive tasks and providing real-time recommendations. This can alleviate the workload of healthcare professionals, improving the quality of care they deliver. Moreover, AI can assist in analyzing vast amounts of data, helping to identify patterns and trends that can be used to enhance patient outcomes and streamline healthcare delivery.

D. Ethical Implications of AI in Healthcare Workforce

The use of AI in healthcare also raises ethical concerns, especially in relation to the healthcare workforce. For instance, healthcare professionals may worry about being replaced by AI algorithms or question the accuracy and reliability of AI-assisted systems. There is also concern about the potential for bias in AI algorithms, which could lead to unequal treatment for certain patient groups. Consequently, it's vital to ensure that ethical considerations are addressed when implementing AI in healthcare, and that healthcare professionals receive appropriate training on how to work effectively and ethically with AI-assisted systems. This will foster a responsible approach to AI integration, maximizing its benefits while minimizing potential risks.

E. Strategies for Managing the Impact of AI on Healthcare Workforce

In order to effectively manage the impact of AI on the healthcare workforce, it is crucial to establish a comprehensive strategy. This may involve reskilling and upskilling healthcare professionals, implementing tailored training programs, and developing ethical guidelines for the responsible use of AI in healthcare. Additionally, ensuring that healthcare professionals possess a clear understanding of the capabilities and limitations of AI-assisted systems will empower them to work effectively alongside these technologies.

Moreover, it is essential to involve healthcare professionals in the development and implementation of AI systems, guaranteeing that their needs and concerns are appropriately addressed. Open communication and collaboration between AI developers, healthcare professionals, and other stakeholders can foster an environment that embraces innovation while maintaining ethical standards.

AI has the potential to significantly transform the healthcare workforce, with both positive and negative implications. Aspects such as automation and job loss, reskilling and upskilling, AI-assisted workflow and efficiency, ethical implications, and strategies for managing the impact of AI on the healthcare workforce should be carefully considered when implementing AI in healthcare. A comprehensive and collaborative strategy is vital to ensure that the benefits of AI are fully realized while minimizing any adverse effects on the healthcare workforce.

8

VIII. AI and Personalized Medicine

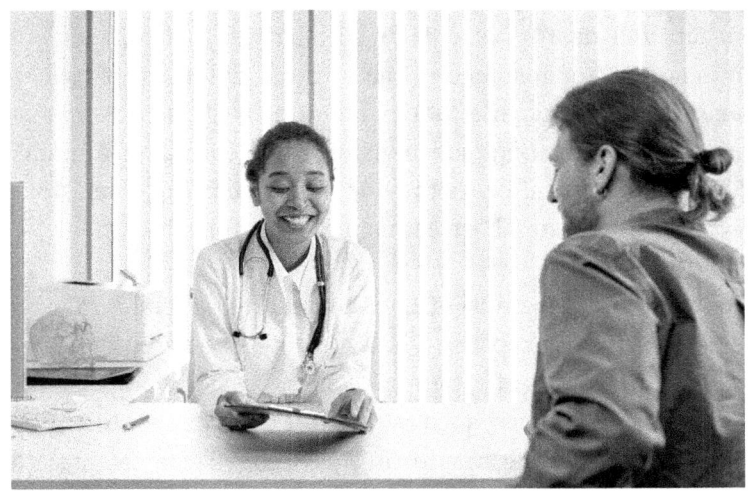

A. Definition of Personalized Medicine

Personalized medicine is a patient-centric approach to healthcare that customizes treatments based on an individual's unique genetic makeup, lifestyle, and environmental factors. This approach seeks to enhance patient outcomes by providing more precise, targeted, and effective treatments tailored to each individual.

B. Role of AI in Personalized Medicine

AI holds significant promise in the realm of personalized medicine, offering powerful tools to analyze vast amounts of data and identify patterns that can be used to predict patient outcomes. For instance, AI algorithms can be employed to analyze patient genetic data, pinpointing genetic markers that may indicate a patient's responsiveness to specific treatments. This can help healthcare providers make informed decisions about the most suitable treatment options for each patient.

Furthermore, AI can be utilized to analyze patient data from electronic health records (EHRs) to detect patterns that may serve as predictors of patient outcomes. By combining insights from various sources, such as genomic data, patient histories, and even real-time monitoring devices, AI can facilitate a more holistic understanding of each patient's unique needs. This in turn enables healthcare professionals to develop more personalized care plans that enhance treatment effectiveness, minimize adverse side effects, and optimize long-term health outcomes.

VIII. AI AND PERSONALIZED MEDICINE

The application of AI in personalized medicine has the potential to revolutionize healthcare by enabling more precise and tailored treatments for each patient. By harnessing the power of AI to analyze complex data, healthcare professionals can make better-informed decisions and ultimately improve patient outcomes across the board.

C. Case Studies

Numerous case studies highlight the application of AI in personalized medicine. For instance, researchers at the University of California, San Francisco, are employing AI to analyze patient data from EHRs, aiming to identify individuals at high risk of developing specific diseases. This approach enables early intervention and tailored prevention strategies. Moreover, researchers at Massachusetts General Hospital are utilizing AI to scrutinize patient genetic data, pinpointing genetic markers that may predict a patient's response to particular treatments, thus facilitating more targeted therapeutic approaches.

D. Challenges and Limitations

WDespite AI's transformative potential in personalized medicine, several challenges and limitations must be addressed. One primary concern is the requirement for vast quantities of data to train AI algorithms effectively. Furthermore, potential biases in AI algorithms may lead to unequal treatment for specific patient groups. Ensuring the accuracy and reliability of AI-assisted systems is also crucial, along with providing adequate training for healthcare professionals to interpret the output of these systems accurately.

AI has the potential to play a significant role in personalized medicine by helping to analyze large amounts of data and identify patterns that can be used to predict patient outcomes. However, it is essential to address challenges and limitations, such as the need for extensive data, potential biases, and the accuracy and reliability of AI-assisted systems. Despite these hurdles, AI's role in personalized medicine is poised to grow increasingly important in the future. Continued research and development will be necessary to unlock the full potential of this transformative technology.

9

IX. The Role of Government and Private Sector in AI in Healthcare

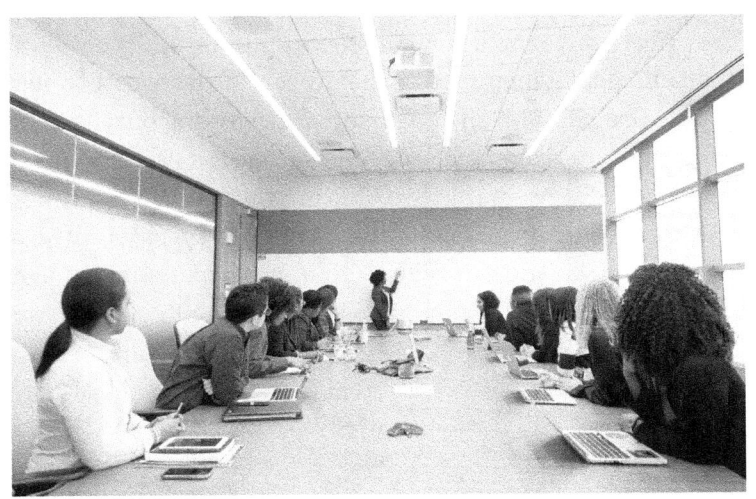

A. Government's Role

The government plays an important role in shaping the development and deployment of AI in healthcare. Government agencies such as the National Institutes of Health (NIH) and the Food and Drug Administration (FDA) fund research on AI in healthcare, and also regulate the use of AI-based medical devices and drugs. Additionally, government policies such as the 21st Century Cures Act and the Affordable Care Act have helped to create an environment that is conducive to the development of AI in healthcare.

B. Private Sector's Role

The private sector also plays an important role in the development and deployment of AI in healthcare. Private companies such as Google, IBM, and Microsoft are investing heavily in AI research and development in healthcare, and are also developing products and services that use AI to improve patient outcomes. Additionally, many hospitals and healthcare systems are also investing in AI, and are using it to improve patient care and reduce costs.

C. Partnership between Government and Private Sector

The partnership between government and the private sector is crucial for the development and deployment of AI in healthcare. Government funding of research and regulation of AI-based medical devices and drugs helps to ensure that these technologies are safe and effective for patients. On the other hand, private sector investment in AI research and development helps to drive innovation and bring new products and services to market.

D. Challenges and Limitations

While the partnership between government and the private sector can help to accelerate the development and deployment of AI in healthcare, there are also several challenges and limitations that need to be considered. One of the main challenges is the need to balance the need for regulation to ensure safety and efficacy with the need for innovation and speed to market. Additionally, there is a need to ensure that AI-based medical devices and drugs are affordable for patients, and that the benefits of these technologies are shared equitably across different population groups.

The partnership between government and the private sector is crucial for the development and deployment of AI in healthcare. Government funding of research and regulation of AI-based medical devices and drugs helps to ensure that these technologies are safe and effective for patients, while private sector investment in AI research and development helps to drive innovation and bring new products and services to market. However, there are also several challenges and limitations that need to be considered, including the need to balance the need for regulation with the need for innovation, and the need to ensure that AI-based medical devices and drugs are affordable for patients. Ongoing dialogue between government and the private sector will be necessary to navigate these challenges and fully realize the potential of AI in healthcare.

10

X. The Impact of AI on Patient Outcomes

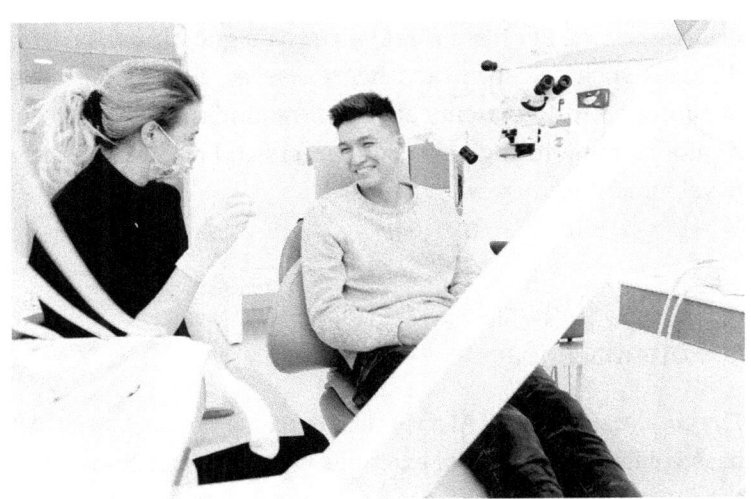

A. Overview

Artificial intelligence (AI) holds immense potential to enhance patient outcomes through more accurate and prompt diagnoses, better patient care, and cost reductions. It is crucial to comprehend AI's current state in healthcare and its prospective influence on patient outcomes.

B. Current Applications

At present, AI is utilized in healthcare for diverse applications, encompassing diagnostic imaging, predictive analytics, and drug discovery. For instance, AI-driven diagnostic tools detect diseases such as cancer and heart disease, while predictive analytics identify patients at risk of readmission. Moreover, AI aids in pinpointing new drug targets and optimizing drug development processes.

C. Potential Impact

The potential impact of AI on patient outcomes is substantial. AI-based diagnostic tools, for example, can significantly enhance the accuracy and speed of disease diagnosis, resulting in earlier treatment and improved patient outcomes. Predictive analytics enable the identification of patients at risk of readmission, facilitating timely interventions and better outcomes. Furthermore, AI contributes to drug development optimization, leading to the discovery of new and more effective treatments for patients.

D. Challenges and Limitations

Although AI offers the promise of significantly improving patient outcomes, several challenges and limitations must be addressed. One primary concern is the need for high-quality data, as AI models' performance is contingent on the data used for training. Additionally, it is essential to ensure that AI-based medical devices and drugs are affordable for patients and that the benefits of these technologies are distributed equitably across diverse population groups.

AI has the potential to significantly improve patient outcomes by providing more accurate and timely diagnoses, enhancing patient care, and reducing costs. However, understanding AI's current state in healthcare and its potential impact on patient outcomes is essential. Ongoing research and development are needed to fully harness AI's potential in healthcare and tackle the challenges and limitations that must be considered.

11

XI. Best Practices for Implementing AI in Healthcare

XI. BEST PRACTICES FOR IMPLEMENTING AI IN HEALTHCARE

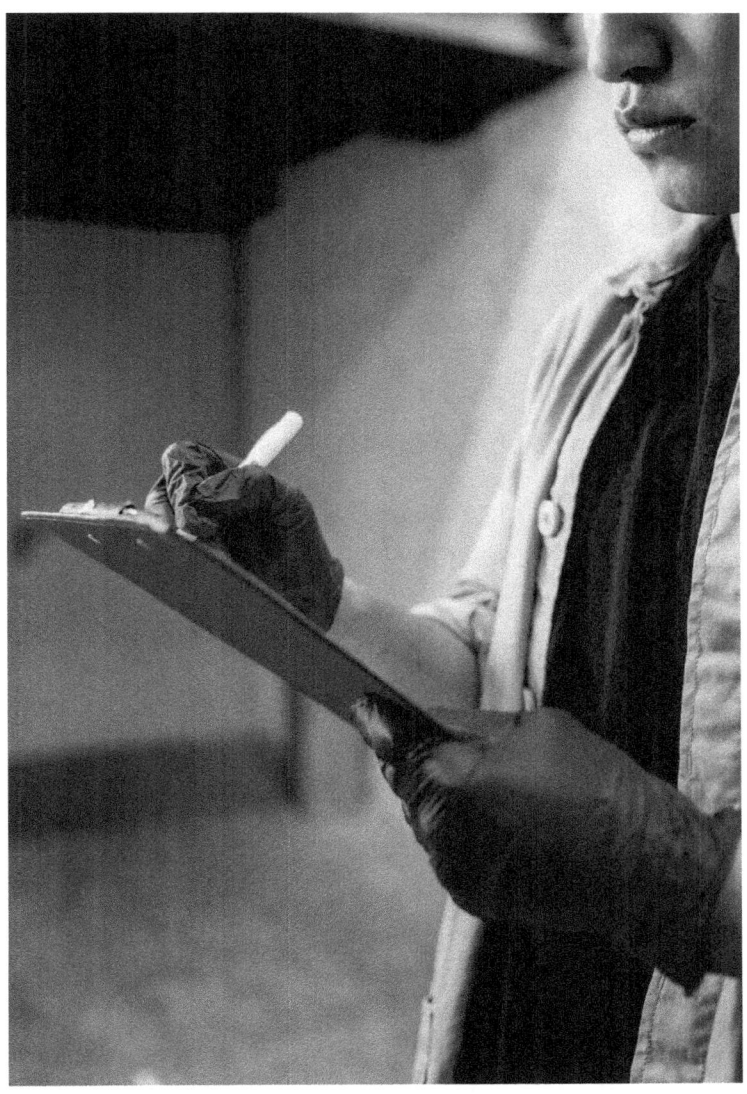

A. Overview

Artificial intelligence (AI) has the potential to significantly improve healthcare delivery and patient outcomes, but the implementation of AI in healthcare requires careful planning and execution. This chapter will provide an overview of best practices for implementing AI in healthcare, including how to identify appropriate use cases, how to select and train AI models, and how to ensure the safety and efficacy of AI-based medical devices and drugs.

B. Identifying Appropriate Use Cases

Identifying appropriate use cases for AI in healthcare is crucial for its successful implementation. This may involve conducting a needs assessment, identifying areas where AI can provide the greatest benefits, and determining the availability of data and resources.

C. Selecting and Training AI Models

Selecting and training AI models that are well-suited to the task at hand is important. This may involve selecting models that have been pre-trained on similar data sets, or training models from scratch using high-quality data.

D. Ensuring Safety and Efficacy

Ensuring the safety and efficacy of AI-based medical devices and drugs is crucial before they are used in clinical practice. This may involve conducting clinical trials, obtaining regulatory approval, and monitoring the performance of AI-based systems over time.

E. Collaboration and Coordination

Implementing AI in healthcare requires collaboration and coordination between different stakeholders, including healthcare providers, researchers, and industry partners. This may involve creating partnerships, sharing data and resources, and establishing governance and oversight mechanisms.

F. Addressing Ethical Considerations

AI in healthcare also raises ethical considerations, such as ensuring fairness, transparency, and accountability in the use of AI systems. Healthcare organizations should establish ethical guidelines for the use of AI in healthcare and ensure that these guidelines are followed in the development and implementation of AI-based systems.

Implementing AI in healthcare requires careful planning and execution. By identifying appropriate use cases, selecting and training AI models, and ensuring the safety and efficacy of AI-based medical devices and drugs, healthcare organizations can maximize the benefits of AI for patients and the healthcare system as a whole. Collaboration and coordination between different stakeholders is also crucial for the successful implementation of AI in healthcare.

XII. Conclusion

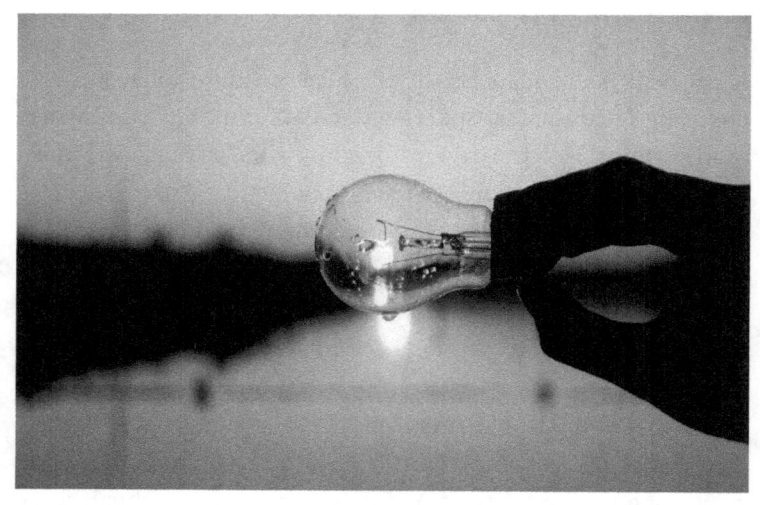

XII. CONCLUSION

A. Summary of key points discussed in the book

This book has discussed the current applications of AI in healthcare, including the use of machine learning for diagnostics and treatment, the use of natural language processing for patient communication, and the use of robotics and assistive technologies in surgery. Additionally, the ethical and legal implications of AI in healthcare were discussed, as well as the challenges and limitations of the technology. The role of government and private sector in AI in healthcare and the impact of AI on patient outcomes were also discussed. Lastly, best practices for implementing AI in healthcare were outlined.

B. Discussion of the future potential of AI in healthcare

The future potential of AI in healthcare is vast, with the technology expected to play an increasingly important role in the diagnosis, treatment, and management of a wide range of medical conditions. AI has the potential to improve the accuracy of medical diagnoses, reduce the cost of healthcare delivery, and improve patient outcomes. In addition, AI can also help to improve the efficiency of healthcare systems and support the delivery of personalized medicine.

C. Call to action for further research and implementation of AI in healthcare

While AI has the potential to revolutionize healthcare, much work is still needed to fully realize this potential. Further research is needed to develop and refine AI algorithms, and to better understand the ethical and legal implications of the technology. Additionally, healthcare organizations must take a strategic approach to the implementation of AI, by identifying appropriate use cases and developing best practices. By continuing to invest in the development and implementation of AI in healthcare, we can help to improve the lives of patients and the healthcare system as a whole.

XIII. Bonus Chapter: AI in Mental Health

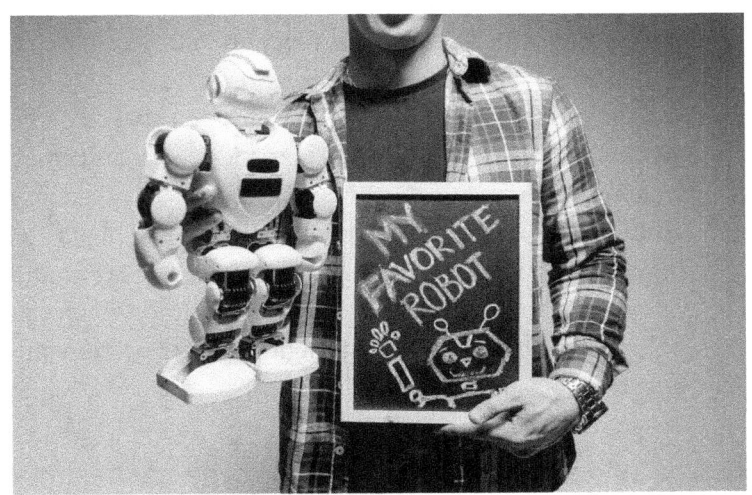

A. Overview of mental health and current challenges

Mental health is a critical aspect of overall health and well-being, yet it is often overlooked and underfunded. Current challenges in mental health care include lack of access to care, stigma, and lack of evidence-based treatment options. AI has the potential to address these challenges by improving access to care, providing personalized treatment, and reducing the burden on healthcare professionals.

B. Applications of AI in mental health

1. **Virtual therapy:** AI-powered chatbots and virtual assistants can provide mental health support and counseling in a convenient, accessible, and anonymous way.
2. **Diagnosis and treatment:** AI can be used to analyze large amounts of data to identify patterns and predict outcomes, which can help mental health professionals to make more accurate diagnoses and personalized treatment plans.
3. **Monitoring and tracking:** AI can be used to track and monitor the progress of patients in real-time, which can help to identify early warning signs of deterioration and ensure timely interventions.

C. Challenges and limitations of AI in mental health

1. **Data privacy and security:** The use of AI in mental health raises significant concerns around data privacy and security, especially given the sensitive nature of mental health data.
2. **Ethical considerations:** AI raises a number of ethical

considerations in mental health, such as the potential for bias and the role of AI in decision-making.
3. **Limited understanding of mental health:** AI's ability to understand and treat mental health is still in its early stages, and more research is needed to fully realize its potential.

AI has the potential to revolutionize the way mental health is diagnosed, treated and monitored. However, in order to fully realize this potential, there is a need for further research, development and implementation of AI in mental health. Additionally, it is crucial to address the ethical, legal and privacy challenges that come with the implementation of AI in mental health. By continuing to invest in the development and implementation of AI in mental health, we can help to improve the lives of patients and the mental health system as a whole.

14

Glossary

Artificial Intelligence (AI): A branch of computer science focused on creating machines that can perform tasks that typically require human intelligence, such as learning, problem-solving, and decision-making.

Algorithm: A set of instructions or rules used by a computer program to solve a problem or perform a task.

Big Data: A term used to describe extremely large data sets that can be analyzed to reveal patterns, trends, and associations.

Clinical Decision Support (CDS): The use of technology to assist healthcare professionals in making clinical decisions, often by providing real-time recommendations based on patient data.

Data Mining: The process of analyzing large data sets to identify patterns, trends, and correlations.

Electronic Health Record (EHR): A digital record of a patient's health history, including medical and treatment history, test results, and diagnoses.

Machine Learning: A subset of AI that focuses on creating algorithms that can learn and improve from data without being explicitly programmed.

Natural Language Processing (NLP): The use of technology to analyze and understand human language, often used in chatbots and virtual assistants.

Personalized Medicine: A medical approach that tailors treatment to the individual patient, taking into account factors such as genetics, lifestyle, and environment.

Predictive Analytics: The use of data, statistical algorithms, and machine learning techniques to identify the likelihood of future outcomes based on historical data.

Robotics: The study and design of robots, machines that can be programmed to perform a variety of tasks.

Supervised Learning: A type of machine learning where an algorithm is trained on labeled data to make predictions or decisions.

Unsupervised Learning: A type of machine learning where an algorithm is trained on unlabeled data to identify patterns and relationships.

Virtual Reality (VR): A technology that creates a simulated environment that can be experienced through a headset or other device. In healthcare, VR can be used for medical training, pain management, and other therapeutic purposes.

Afterword

In this book, we have explored the many ways that AI is being used in healthcare today, and the potential for even more impact in the future. From diagnostics and treatment to patient communication and monitoring, AI has the power to improve the lives of patients and healthcare professionals alike.

However, as with any new technology, there are also challenges and limitations that must be considered. Data privacy and security, ethical considerations, and a lack of understanding of certain areas of healthcare are all issues that must be addressed as we continue to develop and implement AI in healthcare.

It is important to remember that AI is not a panacea for all of healthcare's problems. Rather, it is a tool that can be used to enhance and augment the work of healthcare professionals. By working together, healthcare professionals, researchers, and policymakers can ensure that AI is used to its fullest potential to improve patient outcomes and the healthcare system as a whole.

This book is just the beginning of the conversation about AI in healthcare. We hope it has provided valuable insights and inspiration for further research and implementation of AI in healthcare. Thank you for reading.

Avery

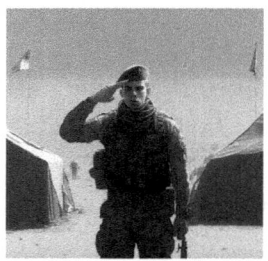

About the Author

Avery Wright is an enigmatic figure who is an author in the fields of AI, Technology, and the Arts. A combat veteran of the US Army, Avery has almost two decades of experience in the IT industry, which has given them a unique perspective on the intersection of technology and society.

As an author, Avery has published a range of books on topics such as the future of AI, the role of drones in modern warfare, and the medicinal properties of mushrooms. Their writing often explores the cutting-edge of technology and how it is changing the world around us. Avery's work is notable for its depth and insight, as well as its ability to make complex topics accessible to a broad audience.

Away from the world of writing, Avery is a private individual who values their privacy. Despite this, they remain a voice in the tech industry and beyond. Whether sharing their thoughts on the latest developments in AI or commenting on the state of the world, Avery's perspective is always worth listening to.

You can connect with me on:
- https://sirexodia.wixsite.com/avery-wright
- https://twitter.com/AveryWrightAI
- https://www.facebook.com/profile.php?id=100089987171726
- https://www.amazon.com/author/averywrightai

Subscribe to my newsletter:
- https://sirexodia.wixsite.com/avery-wright

Also by Avery Wright

Also by Avery Wright
  "Mastering Midjourney AI: The Beginner's Handbook"
  "Chat GPT: A Digital Journey Begins"
  "AI and the Art of Binary"
  "Mycological Marvels: Exploring the Art of AI-Created Mushrooms"
  "AI in Healthcare: How Artificial Intelligence is Transforming Medicine"
  "Transformative Art:: A Journey with Artificial Intelligence"
  "From Predator to Phantom: A Glimpse At Drones"
  "AI and the Future of Humanity"
  "The Tao of Inner Peace"
  "Taoism Unleashed: Advanced Concepts for Deepening Your Practice"
  "The Knife's Edge:: A View on the Ultra Rich and their Motivations"
  "Defending the Skies: The Rise of Unidentified Aerial Phenomena and the Battle for Airspace Dominance"
  "Mastering the Board: The Power of Pawns in Chess"
  "The Brain in the Machine: Understanding the Inner Workings of Artificial Intelligence"
  "Healing with Fungi: The Science of Medicinal Mushrooms"
  "Chat GPT: ChatGPT Explores the World: Conversations Across Cultures"
  "Chat GPT: Unleashing ChatGPT's Power: Navigating the Digital Realm"

Avery Wright's work spans a range of topics, from the cutting-edge of AI and technology to the ancient practice of Taoism and the art of chess. Their books are notable for their depth, insight, and ability to make complex topics accessible to a broad audience. With almost two decades of experience in the IT field and a background as a combat veteran, Avery brings a unique perspective to their writing that is both informative and thought-provoking. Whether you are interested in exploring the frontiers of technology or deepening your understanding of the human experience, Avery's books are a must-read.

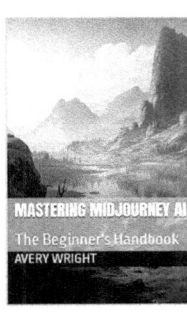

Mastering Midjourney AI - The Beginner's Handbook

Mastering Midjourney AI: The Beginner's Handbook is a comprehensive guide for beginners looking to learn about the Midjourney AI platform and how to use it for image generation. The book covers a range of topics, including understanding Midjourney AI's parameters and settings, using URLs for image inspiration, adjusting image quality, and more.
https://www.amazon.com/dp/B0BV8PGDXT

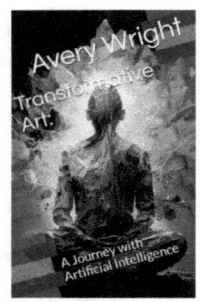

Transformative Art - A Journey with Artificial Intelligence

Transformative Art: A Journey with AI is a visually stunning and thought-provoking book that explores the intersection of artificial intelligence and the world of art. The book features breathtaking images of futuristic cities, technology, vehicles, robots, flying ships, conceptual art, abstract art, and unique pieces, all within the context of transformative art. Each chapter begins with a powerful quote that sets the tone for a deep dive into the themes of perception, change, reflection, risk-taking, emotional connection, the journey within, and the universal language of art. The book is written by Avery Wright, a talented author with a passion for exploring the ways in which technology is changing our lives and our world. This book is a must-read for anyone interested in the intersection of art, technology, and the human experience. https://www.amazon.com/dp/B0BTWNYLJD

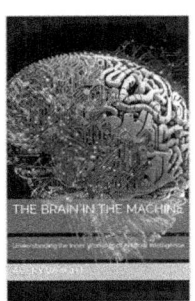

The Brain in the Machine: Understanding the Inner Workings of Artificial Intelligence (Mastering AI)

"The Brain in the Machine: Understanding the Inner Workings of Artificial Intelligence" provides a comprehensive and accessible introduction to the field of artificial intelligence. From the history of AI to the latest advances in deep learning, natural language processing, and computer vision, this book covers a wide range of topics to help readers understand the inner workings of AI. With a focus on the practical applications of AI, this book is an ideal resource for students, researchers, and practitioners in the field.
https://www.amazon.com/dp/B0BW6FGRTK

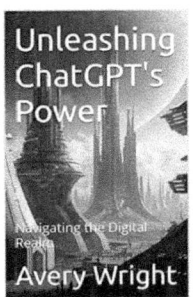

Unleashing ChatGPT's Power: Navigating the Digital Realm

"Unleashing ChatGPT's Power: Navigating the Digital Realm" explores the complex and sophisticated technology behind one of the most innovative and exciting technological advancements of our time. Through in-depth discussions of the underlying technology that powers ChatGPT, its ability to process natural language, and its expanding knowledge base, readers will gain a deeper understanding of the ways in which artificial intelligence and natural language processing are shaping the future of society.
https://www.amazon.com/dp/B0BVSYQ77H

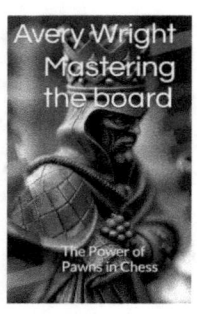

Mastering the board: The Power of Pawns in Chess (Chess Masterclass Series)
This book delves into the often overlooked, yet incredibly important aspect of the game of chess - the pawns. From its introduction to the various strategies and techniques for using pawns effectively, this book is designed to provide a comprehensive guide to understanding the power of pawns in chess. Whether you are a beginner or an experienced player, this book will provide valuable insights and techniques that you can use to improve your pawn play and overall chess game.

https://www.amazon.com/dp/B0BW8HB1PN

www.ingramcontent.com/pod-product-compliance
Lightning Source LLC
Chambersburg PA
CBHW050253220526
45465CB00002B/667